DASH Diet

Complete Dash Diet Weight Loss Cookbook for, Lower Blood Pressure, Lower Cholesterol, and Great Recipes

Introduction

I want to thank you and congratulate you for downloading the book, *"DASH Diet: Complete Dash Diet Weight Loss Cookbook for, Lower Blood Pressure, Lower Cholesterol, and Great Recipes"*.

This book has lots of actionable information that will help you to follow the DASH diet to lose weight, lower blood pressure and cholesterol.

With the world increasingly becoming more plagued by heart disease, type 2 diabetes, hypertension, cancer, obesity and other lifestyle related complications, it is easy for the masses to lose hope of ever getting to old age. So what are you to do to increase your odds of defeating or even preventing some of these health complications?

Well, the secret is in changing our way of life e.g. changing our eating and exercise habits. Would it not be great if we could have a diet that could reduce the effects of various diseases through lowering blood pressure, keeping your heart healthy through lowering cholesterol and at the same time helping you lose weight?

Obviously, life would be a lot better if we could naturally prime our bodies in a way that ensures we avoid heart disease, diabetes, hypertension and a host of other health complications. And that's where the DASH diet comes in!

If you are wondering what the diet is all about, this book will give you strategies that will set you up on the path massive success when dealing with these and other related complications. It will also give you sample recipes as well as a meal plan to hold you by the hand in your journey to losing weight, reducing blood pressure and cholesterol as well as other complications.

FREE BONUS VIDEO BELLOW

https://www.youtube.com/watch?v=RgUwTiRXof8

Thanks again for downloading this book. I hope you enjoy it!

Table of Contents

Before we can start discussing the specifics of what to do to follow a DASH diet, it is important to start by building an understanding of what the diet is and what it is all about. Let's begin.

DASH Diet: A Comprehensive Overview

What Is It?

The DASH diet, which stands for Dietary Approaches to Stop Hypertension, is a diet that was first created with the aim of reducing high blood pressure/ hypertension. The diet is essentially designed to minimize the intake of saturated fats, cholesterol and total fats while monitoring the intake of sweets, red meats, snacks, and beverages with added sugars.

So how is the diet able to control hypertension anyway?

Well, it does that by greatly limiting the intake of sodium, found in salt.

And how is salt involved in all blood pressure balance or imbalance?

Simple; salts greatly affect the body's ability to hold more water, a phenomenon that ultimately increases blood pressure, which puts up more pressure on your brain, arteries as well as the heart.

Let me explain that.

The kidneys have a role to filter blood to get rid of impurities, which are then removed with urine. They (kidneys) draw any excess water from the bloodstream through osmosis through a pretty delicate sodium-potassium balance in a bid to collect water from the cells into the bladder. When your sodium intake is high (through higher salt intake for instance), this results to increased sodium concentrations in the bloodstream, a phenomenon that ends up messing up with the delicate sodium-potassium balance that we've just mentioned. As a result, your kidneys have a harder time excreting the excess water, a phenomenon that brings a strain in your blood vessels (especially those leading to the kidneys). The excess pressure can over time result to damage of the kidneys if it progresses to kidney disease. Moreover, a high blood pressure can cause damage to your arteries because this excess blood pressure puts some extra strain on the walls of your arteries. Any attempts by your body to correct the problem only end up putting you at a higher risk of complications. For instance, it may respond by making the walls stronger and thicker but this only makes the insides a lot smaller resulting to greater blood pressure, which may even damage the arteries leading to your heart (e.g. the arteries might burst or the pressure might cause a heart attack). Worse still, a higher blood pressure might end up predisposing you to a stroke.

You follow a DASH diet (which suggests you reduce your intake of both natural and added salts) to help reduce the probability of developing high blood pressure (less 2000mg of sodium enriched food is sufficient to lower your blood pressure in as little as 2 weeks although you shouldn't discontinue your medication without consulting with your doctor).

Because of its valuable composition, the diet realized some extra benefits such as weight loss and several others. Further research was then done and some modifications made to make it even more effective for weight loss and fighting hypertension. This is where the 2 forms of DASH diet come in i.e.

✓ The standard DASH diet: This one calls for taking just 2500mg of sodium per day.

✓ Low sodium DASH diet: In this case, you aim for between 1500-1700mg of sodium per day. It is suited for those over 50 years and is based on the US National Heart Association 1700mg limit.

One interesting bit about the diet is that you can take as many calories as you want, as long as you maintain your sodium levels within the two limits set above. In the DASH diet, you have the option of choosing a diet option that will work best for you in accordance to your weight maintenance or weight loss goals. You can choose a plan that either provides 3100, 2600, 2000, 1600 or 1,200 calories in a day.

So what should you eat while on a DASH diet?

What To Eat

Generally, the diet recommends a high intake of certain foods that ensure you get a good supply of minerals like potassium, calcium and magnesium as well as fiber.

- Fruits

- Low fat milk products

- Poultry

- Veggies

- Whole grains

- Fish

- Nuts

Eating whole grains, veggies and fruits gives you more antioxidants as well as phytonutrients, which can greatly help you to reduce the chances of developing diabetes, heart disease as well as cancer. Antioxidants and phytonutrients are very effective for promoting weight loss. Make sure to take them fresh and organic; not supplements.

To sum everything up, the diet requires the following:

✓ Eat more fruits, low fat dairy and vegetables while minimizing intake of processed cheese given that just 2 ounces contain as much as 600mg of sodium.

✓ Cut back on foods, which are high in trans fats, cholesterol and saturated fats

✓ Eat more fish, whole grain foods, nuts and poultry and limiting sweets, red meats, sodium and sugary drinks. A hotdog has up to 460mg of sodium while a tablespoon of soy sauce contains up to 900mg of sodium and a serving of frozen pizza (with the meat and veggies) has up to 982mg of sodium.

✓ Don't take more than 2300mg of sodium or sodium enriched food in a day; a tablespoon of salt has about

2300mg of sodium while a hamburger has around 600mg of sodium.

Note: Don't just substitute salt with the most available item; it could be harmful to you. For instance, some might contain potassium chloride, which has been reported to cause complications for those suffering from cancer and diabetes. You don't have to rely on substitutes to lower your salt intake. For instance, you can take more spices and herbs to season your food e.g. black pepper, ginger, turmeric, cinnamon, garlic etc.

To make this easy for you to follow, you can refer to the guidelines below:

Generally, the daily recommendations of the DASH diet are:

- ✓ 7 to 8 servings of whole grain

- ✓ 2 to 3 servings of fat free or low fat dairy

- ✓ 2 servings (or less) of fish, lean meats and poultry

- ✓ 4 to 5 servings of vegetables and fruit

- ✓ And on a weekly perspective- 3 to 5 servings of nuts, legumes and seeds and less than 5 servings of sweets

- ✓ 2-3 servings of fats and oils

This might sound like huge portions but wait until you know what exactly a serving is in a 'normal' world. Represented by the different types of foods, a serving is:

- ✓ ½ cup of cooked pasta or rice

- ✓ 1 slice of bread

- ✓ 1 cup of raw fruit or vegetables

- ✓ ½ cup of cooked fruit or veggies

- ✓ Eight ounces of milk

- ✓ One teaspoon of olive oil /or just any other type of oil

- ✓ 3 ounces of cooked meat

- ✓ 3 ounces of tofu

Approximately, this diet gets 55% of its calories from carbs, 27% from total fats and 6% from saturated fats, 18% from proteins whereas fiber is 30 grams and cholesterol limited to 150mg.

Even with the above description, you might still have a hard time reducing how much salt you take. Here are some great ideas to make it easy for you:

- If you are taking fish, it is best to opt for the boiled or steamed versions then season with natural spices and herbs. Make sure not to opt for those with added preservatives and salts!

- Different condiments tend to be high in sodium. For instance, sauces often have added salts so if you are ordering veggies, it is best to avoid a situation where you will need to use sauce. For instance, you can take steamed veggies. You will find more salt in ketchup, mustard and pickles.

- It is best to avoid buying foods or ingredients containing any salts

What about fats; how do you lower your intake of saturated fats and cholesterol to help fight off heart disease? Here are some ideas:

- Insist on eating foods cooked through friendly methods like grilling, baking, grilling, roasting, broiling, poaching and stir frying.

- Trim fat from poultry, fish and red meat and ensure to take small servings

- Reduce your reliance on salad dressings and only take vinegar or oil

With that understanding, let's now discuss how to follow the diet in the remaining part of the book. For starters, it is important to appreciate that the typical DASH diet has 2 phases:

The DASH Diet In Action

Phase 1: Day 1-14: Reducing Your Waistline

The first 2 weeks entail eliminating whole grains, which tend to be high in carbohydrates (this spikes blood sugar). Instead, you eat more of foods that have natural sugars like Greek yogurt, skim milk and various other low fat dairy products. Why should you opt for that? Well, because these two are filling and can help you to reduce unnecessary cravings.

Here is a detailed explanation of **what to eat**:

Plenty of veggies i.e. parsley, broccoli, kales, spinach or collard greens

4-5 servings of lentils/beans per week

2-3 servings of low fat dairy e.g. a cup of skim milk or low fat yogurt

6 ounces of lean meat, fish or poultry per day

Tomatoes, cucumbers, pepper, squash etc.-these can help reduce pressure and keep cravings at bay

Avocadoes tossed in canola, olive or nut oils

Fatty fish e.g. mackerel, tuna, salmon, as well as nuts and seeds

As you do this, make sure to avoid the following:

Grains and grain products like rice, wheat flour, pasta, cakes etc.

High fructose or fresh fruit

Alcoholic beverages

Foods fried in butter

Fat free cheese (contains up to 95% sodium!)

Starchy veggies like potatoes, corn, and winter squash

Phase 2

When you get to week 2, you can start introducing some starchy foods then increase your intake of whole grains as well as low fat foods. To put this into perspective, here is what you can eat and what you ought to avoid:

What to eat:

Quinoa

Baked fish

Skim milk

Baby carrots

Cashews

4-6 ounces of berries

Lean cuts of turkey

1-2 light cheese wedges for mid-morning snack

Brown rice

Veggies e.g. broccoli, kales, asparagus and lettuce

Blueberry light yogurt for your afternoon snacks

Whole wheat pasta

Sugar free strawberry Jello-O cup for your desserts

What not to eat

Trans fat margarine

Salted canned tomatoes

Sweetened applesauce

High sodium soy sauce as well as teriyaki sauce

High sodium beef or vegetable broth

Bleached as well as processed wheat flour

Instant oatmeal

High calorie frozen desserts e.g. juice bars

Phase 2's duration is dependent on your weight or blood pressure.

Let's take the discussion a bit further where we will be discussing how to build a perfect meal plan while you are on a DASH diet.

How To Make The Perfect Meal Plan

Considering the DASH diet has a few variations in accordance to calorie requirement, the meal plans might be a bit different.

But here are **general DASH diet tips regardless of the meal plan**:

For the condiments

Use fat free or low fat condiments and only a half of your usual serving of salad dressing, butter or margarine. Find other better alternatives to salt and only use it when it is a matter of life and death. One of the alternatives could be low sodium salt alternative, which just tastes the same as regular table salt but uses potassium instead of sodium as the major ingredient. But make sure you check with your doctor first before using an alternative.

Go crazy on veggies

Include a serving of veggies at dinner and at lunch. It doesn't matter what you are eating; just throw in some kale or veggies but don't overdo it if you are trying to lose weight (veggies do contain carbs). Make sure to also include generous amounts of dry beans to your diet.

Meat

Limit your meat intake to 6 ounces in a day and try and make some meals vegetarian. Processed meats contain hidden sodium as they are preserved and seasoned with salt so keep your meat grass fed and fresh.

Watch out!

Always read food labels so that you can choose those foods that have lower quantities of sodium. Also try and avoid processed foods as they contain more salt than you think- for instance, nearly 80% of the salt consumed in just North America comes from foods such as frozen entrees, deli meats, canned soups, pickles and condiments.

Keep it low

In anytime that you would use cream or full fat, use skim or low fat dairy products. These contain less fat hence a bit heart friendly.

Fruit up

Use fruit as a snack or add a serving of fruit to your meals. Dried and canned fruits are flexible to use but first make sure they don't contain any added sugars.

Snacking

Instead of the usual snacking on sweets or chips, snack on raisins, unsalted nuts or pretzels, plain unsalted popcorn with no butter and raw veggies.

Meal Planning Based On Different Caloric Requirements

When you are equipped with the right tools, it will be so easy to keep on the DASH diet track. Different people have different caloric needs- depending on how physically active you are. Normally, males need more calories than females (not to sound sexist or anything). For instance, a male at the age between 19 to 30 and is not physically active will require 2400 calories daily (2600-3000 if active) while a female who is also not physically active will require 2000 calories in a day (2000-2400 if active).

In the DASH diet, you can choose a meal plan that has 1600, 2000 or 2600 calories in a day.

Note: regardless of the calorie count, aim to eat the meals throughout the day instead of at the same time- for instance, if you will be having a banana and a whole wheat bagel for breakfast, you can eat the banana first then after a few hours eat the bagel. Distribute your meals to make a total of at least 6 meals in a day.

Meal Plan For 1600 Calories

If your calorie requirement is 1600 daily, you can adopt the following DASH diet eating style:

Weekly oils: 2 teaspoons

Fruits: have 2 cups in a day

Daily low fat or fat free milk and dairy: 2 to 3 cups

Daily lean poultry, meat and fish: 3 to 6 ounces

Daily legumes, seeds and nuts: 3 to 4 times

Daily veggies: have 1 ½ to 2 cups

Alcohol, salt and sweets: use sparingly

Daily whole grains: 6 ounces

Example (approximately 1600 calories)

Breakfast

1 medium banana

1 whole-wheat bagel

1 cup fat-free milk

2 tablespoons peanut butter

Lunch

1 medium apple

Turkey sandwich

1 cup fat-free milk

½ cup baby carrots

Dinner

½ cup green beans

Baked chicken breast

1 cup salad

1 cup brown rice pilaf

Snacks

1 cup fresh seasonal fruit

1 cup fat-free yogurt

Meal Plan For 2000 Calories

Daily veggies: have 2 to 2 ½ cups

Alcohol, salt and sweets: use sparingly

Fruits: have 2 to 2 ½ cups in a day

Daily low fat or fat free milk and dairy: 2 to 3 cups

Daily lean poultry, meat and fish: 6 or less ounces

Daily legumes, seeds and nuts: 4 to 5 times

Daily whole grains: 6 to 8 ounces

Weekly oils: 2 to 3 teaspoons

Example (approximately 2000 calories)

Breakfast

1 cup fat-free milk

2 tablespoons peanut butter

1 medium banana

1 whole-wheat bagel

Lunch

½ cup baby carrots

Turkey sandwich

1 cup fat-free milk

1 medium apple

Dinner

1 cup salad

Baked chicken breast

½ cup green beans

1 cup fresh seasonal fruit

1 cup brown rice pilaf

Snacks

1 cup fat-free yogurt

1 cup fresh seasonal fruit

½ cup sliced cucumbers

Meal Plan For 2600 Calories

Alcohol, salt and sweets: use sparingly

Daily whole grains: 10 to 11 ounces

Fruits: have 2 ½ to 3 cups in a day

Daily low fat or fat free milk and dairy: 3 cups

Daily lean poultry, meat and fish: 6 ounces

Daily legumes, seeds and nuts: 1 portion

Daily veggies: have 2 ½ to 3 cups

Weekly oils: 2 to 3 teaspoons

Example (approximately 2600 calories)

Breakfast

1 whole-wheat bagel

4 ounces of orange juice

1 medium banana

1 ounce bran flakes with 1 cup of fat-free milk

2 tablespoons peanut butter

Lunch

½ cup baby carrots

1 ounce whole grain crackers

1 medium apple

1 cup fat-free milk

Turkey sandwich

Dinner

1 cup salad

½ cup green beans

1 small dinner roll

Baked chicken breast

1 cup brown rice pilaf

Snacks

1 cup fat-free yogurt with ½ a cup of frozen berries and ¼ cup of granola

1 cup of fresh seasonal fruit

½ cup of sliced cucumbers

Other Strategies To Maximize Fat Loss, Lower Blood Pressure And Cholesterol

1> Drink tea

Drinking tea can help reduce hypertension- However, keep in mind that some teas are more effective than others while others, especially the caffeinated ones, may heighten blood pressure in the short term. The ones best for reducing blood pressure are:

Hibiscus tea: The tea is naturally sweet (but you can add honey or stevia if you like) and you can make it and use it in place of water for about 3 cups of some fluid.

Hawthorn tea: this plant has been used to battle heart disease for as long as back in the 1st century. 3 cups a day is enough.

Gotu kola tea: This is another great tea, which is specifically great at combating venous insufficiency. This tea is believed to assist in maintaining connective tissue thereby strengthening veins and improving circulation. Again, 3 cups a day is the recommendation for this tea.

Green tea and oolong: these teas can be really beneficial at reducing hypertension. In fact, one study showed that drinking at least 1 ½ to 2 ½ cups of green tea or oolong reduces the risk of having high blood pressure by 46%.

2> Exercise

Exercise is one of the best and effective ways to reduce blood pressure, lower cholesterol and lose weight. Exercise works well in reducing blood pressure through reducing insulin levels by depletion of glucose.

A well planned routine inclusive of sprint burst-type exercises, aerobics and strength training can help greatly in reducing both your blood pressure and insulin levels. You will want to have someone to monitor your progress and supervise you throughout your program to make sure you are doing it correctly. You can dedicate an hour a day to do this. Make sure to start slowly and work your way upwards though.

3> If you do, quit smoking

Quitting smoking can improve your HDL (high density lipoprotein- or the good cholesterol) levels.

Picture this; just 20 minutes after you quit the smokes, your heart rate and your blood pressure decreases and within a year, your risk of having heart disease is half of that of a smoker. Within about 15 years, your risk is just like that of the one who has never smoked.

4> Eat your own meals

You should avoid all fast food restaurants and limit eating restaurant food. First of all, fast food makes you fat (high in simple carb and bad fats), no questions asked. Second, eating out limits your chances of tracking what you are eating. If you check out the nutritional info of meals in chain restaurant websites, you will be shocked; you can exceed your sodium limit in only a single meal without knowing it. The only safety assured in eating out is asking for foods that are not pre seasoned such as grilled fish and salads. Or better yet, just cook your own meals with natural ingredients to make sure that what you eat doesn't exceed your limits.

5> Manage your stress

People who are psychologically stressed (especially if they have major hostility, depression and/ or anger) may be at a higher risk of heart disease. As much as stress has not been fully proved to cause chronic blood pressure, episodes of stress have the ability to cause a temporary raise in hypertension.

Stress can also lead to weight gain through the production of the hormone cortisol, which heightens cravings. You can manage your stress through a series of meditation and yoga techniques, finding distractions or talking to someone about it.

With that in mind, the next chapter will introduce some DASH diet recipes to get you started.

Sample DASH Recipes

Breakfast

Apple spice baked oatmeal

Nutrition Information: 160 calories, 6 g total fat, 22 g carbohydrates, 6 g protein, 150 mg sodium, 30 mg potassium

Servings: 9

Ingredients

¼ teaspoon salt

2 tablespoons oil

1 teaspoon baking powder

1 egg- beaten

1 teaspoon cinnamon

1 ½ cups non-fat or 1% milk

1 teaspoon vanilla

1 apple- chopped (about 1 ½ cups)

2 cups rolled oats

½ cup applesauce- sweetened

Topping

2 tablespoons chopped nuts

2 tablespoons brown sugar

Instructions

Preheat your oven to 375 degrees F and spray or lightly oil a baking pan (8 x 8 inch).

Combine the apple sauce, vanilla, egg, oil and milk in a bowl.

Add in the apple. Mix the baking powder, cinnamon, rolled oats and salt in another bowl.

Add this mixture to the liquid ingredients and combine well.

Pour the combined mixture into the baking dish and let it bake for 25 minutes. Take out of the oven and sprinkle with nuts and brown sugar.

Add it back to the oven and let it broil for about 3 to 4 minutes, until the top appears browned and the sugar is bubbling- make sure it doesn't burn.

Cut your meal into nine pieces of 2.5 by 2.5 inch squares and serve while warm. Ensure you refrigerate any leftovers within 2 hours.

Note: Add a glass of low fat milk to the meal to make it really dash. You can substitute the apple for other types of fruit-just get creative- e.g. bananas, pears, blueberries, etc.

Chocolate Smoothie With Avocado And Banana

Nutritional info: 252 calories, 822 milligrams potassium, 102 milligrams sodium, 12 grams fat, 11 grams proteins, 33 grams Carbs

Servings: 2

Ingredients

½ avocado- pitted and peeled

2 individual packets Splenda

1 medium banana- peeled

2 cups vanilla soy milk

¼ cup unsweetened cocoa powder

Instructions

Add all ingredients to a blender and run the blender until smooth. Serve right away and enjoy!

Easy Middle Eastern Hummus Wrap

Servings: 1

Nutritional info: 302 calories, 12.13g total fat, 12.64g protein, 557.12mg Sodium, 39.9g total carbs

Ingredients

½ teaspoon ground black pepper

1 whole-wheat tortilla (8-inch)

½ teaspoon lemon zest

¼ whole long English cucumber, thinly sliced

1/3 cup hummus

¼ medium red onion, thinly sliced

1 cup baby lettuce mix

8 leaf fresh mint leaves

1 teaspoon 100% lemon juice

1 plum tomato, thinly sliced

Instructions

Spread the hummus all over the tortilla and top it with the rest of the ingredients. Roll up the tortilla tightly and enjoy.

Note: You can use any other type of healthy vegetables in substitute for the ones suggested. You can also use any type of flavoured hummus of your choice.

Zucchini Bread

Nutritional info: Calories 141, 5g total fat, 103 mg sodium, 4g protein, 22g carbs

Servings: 18 (2 loaves)

Ingredients

3 teaspoons ground cinnamon

½ cup sugar

1 ¼ cups whole-wheat (whole-meal) flour

1 teaspoon baking powder

¼ cup canola oil

½ cup chopped walnuts

6 egg whites

2 cups shredded zucchini

2 teaspoons vanilla extract

½ cup unsweetened applesauce

1 teaspoon baking soda

1 ½ cups crushed, unsweetened pineapple

1 ¼ cups of all-purpose (plain) flour

Instructions

Preheat your oven to 350 degrees F and lightly coat 2 9 x 5 inch loaf pans using cooking spray.

Add the canola oil, sugar, egg whites, applesauce and vanilla to a large bowl. Use an electric mixture to combine the ingredients on a low speed until foamy and thick.

Stir together the flours in a small bowl and set ½ a cup aside. Add in the baking soda, cinnamon and baking powder to the bowl of flour.

Add the flours to the egg white mixture and beat using the electric mixer on the medium setting.

When it is well blended, add in the zucchini, pineapple and walnuts and stir until they combine.

Use the ½ cup of flour you set aside to adjust the batter's consistency- it should not be runny, just about thick.

Pour the batter equally into the 2 prepared pans and add them to the preheated oven.

Bake for about 50 minutes or until when a toothpick is inserted, it comes out clean.

Allow the bread to cool on a wire rack in the pans for about 10 minutes. Take the loves out of the pan and let them cool completely on the rack. Cut both loaves into 9 1 inch slices and enjoy.

Lunch Recipes

Salmon and Edamame Cakes

Nutritional info: 267 calories, 1g fat, 1g fiber, 166mg sodium, 21g proteins

Servings: 4

Ingredients

¼ cup panko (Japanese-style bread crumbs) - preferably whole wheat panko

2 large egg whites

1 clove garlic- crushed through a press

1 tablespoon peeled then minced fresh ginger

Lime wedges- for serving

Canola oil in a pump sprayer

1 scallion finely chopped- white and green parts

1 tablespoon of finely chopped fresh cilantro

2 cups of flaked cooked salmon (about 13 ounces)

½ cup thawed frozen edamame

Instructions

Mix the panko, ginger, cilantro, salmon, egg whites, scallion and garlic in a medium bowl.

Add in the edamame. Form 4 3½ inch wide cakes from the mixture.

Transfer the cakes onto a waxed paper lined plate and put it into the refrigerator for about 15 to 30 minutes.

Use oil to spray a non stick skillet (large) and heat it over medium heat. Add in the cakes of salmon and cook them for about 3 to 4 until their underside is browned.

Flip them over and cook for another 3 to 4 minutes until the underside is also browned. Serve while hot with the wedges of lime.

Cod With Lemon And Capers

Nutritional info: 168 Calories, total fat 4g, 2g total carbohydrates, Protein 31g, 203mg Sodium

Servings: 4

Ingredients

1 tablespoon all-purpose (plain) flour

1 cup hot tap water

2 lemons

4 cod fillets- each 6 ounces

4 teaspoons capers, rinsed and drained

1 teaspoon bouillon granules, low-sodium (chicken-flavored)

1 tablespoon soft butter

Instructions

Preheat your oven to 350 degrees F.

Use cooking spray to spray 4 squares of foil. Take each cod fillet and place it on the oiled foil squares.

Cut one lemon into two and squeeze out the juice from one half all over the fish and the other half cut it into thin slices and place it on top of the fish.

Seal the foil. Place the prepared fish in the preheated oven and bake for about 20 minutes until the fish is opaque when you test it with the tip of your knife.

As the fish is cooking, take the other lemon and remove the peel (don't slice off the pith, just the peel).

Slice the peel into a quarter inch (width) stripes. Add the chicken bouillon and the hot tap water in a small bowl. Stir until the granules dissolve and set aside.

Mix the flour and butter in another small bowl and transfer to a heavy saucepan.

Place it over moderate heat and stir until the flour-butter mixture melts.

Add in the bullion to the flour mixture and continue stirring until its thick. Add in the capers and take off from heat. Serve it over the fish with the lemon peel as garnish.

Leafy Rotisserie Chicken Salad With Tarragon Dressing

Nutritional info: 362 calories, 39.16g total carbs, 10.59g total fat, 64.91mg sodium, 26.38g protein

Servings: 2 cups

Ingredients

1 cup English Cucumber- thinly sliced

3 tablespoons pine nuts

½ medium red onion - thinly sliced

1 tablespoon extra-virgin olive oil

6 cups Mesclun Salad Mix

1/3 cup White Balsamic Vinegar

15 ounces canned white beans

1 1/3 cups Cooked Chicken Breast -chopped

¾ teaspoon ground black pepper

2 garlic clove

2 tablespoon tarragon, fresh- divided

12 Grapes thinly sliced (Red or Green)

Instructions

Add the vinegar, garlic, ½ cup of the beans, oil and a tablespoon of the tarragon to the blender and cover then blend to combine.

Arrange all the greens on a large platter and top it with the remaining beans, chicken, cucumber, pepper, onion, grapes, nuts and the rest of the tarragon.

Serve the prepared dressing on the side.

African Sweet Potato & Chicken Stew

Nutritional info: 615 calories, 24.0g fat, 66.0g carbohydrates, 35.0 g protein, 457 mg sodium

Servings: 4

Ingredients

2 teaspoons ground coriander- divided

¾ teaspoon salt- divided

2 tablespoons extra-virgin olive oil- divided

1 large sweet potato (about 1 pound), peeled and cubed (½-inch)

1½ cups water

1 large onion, halved and sliced

1 28-ounce can of chopped tomatoes with salt added (see Tip), reserve juice

1 cup whole-wheat couscous

¼ cup of smooth natural peanut butter

2 tablespoons lime juice- divided

1 pound boneless, skinless chicken thighs- trimmed

¼ teaspoon cayenne pepper or ½ teaspoon crushed red pepper

1 cup chopped cilantro

1 tablespoon grated fresh ginger

Instructions

Cut the chicken into small bite sized pieces and sprinkle them with a tablespoon of coriander and ½ a teaspoon of salt.

Add oil to a large non stick skillet and place it over medium high heat.

Once it heats, add in the chicken and cook as you stir until it is browned all around for about 4 minutes.

Transfer the browned chicken to a plate. Add the remaining tablespoon of oil, ginger and onion to the pan and cook as you stir for 3 to 5 minutes until everything is lightly browned.

Add in the sweet potato, peanut butter, cayenne (or red pepper- crushed), tomatoes with their juices, ¼ teaspoon of salt, a tablespoon of lime juice and 1 teaspoon of coriander.

Let it boil then lower the heat to allow it to simmer then cover.

Cook as you stir on occasion for 14 to 16 minutes until the sweet potato is tender.

Add back the chicken with any accumulated juices to the pan and cook for two more minutes until it is heated all through.

In the meantime, add water to a medium sauce pan and bring it to a boil. Add in a tablespoon of lime and the couscous.

Cover then take off heat and allow it to stand for 5 minutes. Fluff it using a fork and stir in the cilantro. Serve the stew on top of the couscous.

Tip: For the best tomato flavor with little to no added sodium, read the labels and compare; choose the ones with 190mg of sodium or less per half a cup serving.

Dinner Recipes

Garlic Mashed Potatoes

Nutritional info: 145 Calories, 7 milligrams sodium, 7 grams fat, 19 grams Carbs, 2 grams proteins

Servings: 8

Ingredients

1 teaspoon salt-free seasoning blend

¼ cup olive oil

½ teaspoon freshly ground black pepper

6 cloves garlic- peeled

2 pounds of all-purpose red/ gold potatoes- scrubbed and cut into large chunks

Instructions

Place the peeled garlic cloves and the potato chunks into a large saucepan.

Cover it with some cold water and let it boil.

Lower the heat when it boils and let it simmer until when pierced with a fork, the potatoes are tender, for about 25 minutes.

Take off from heat and drain out the liquid from the potatoes making sure to reserve ¾ of that liquid.

Add in the salt free seasoning blend, reserved cooking liquid, olive oil and pepper into the potatoes.

Use a large fork or a potato masher to mash them and season with some pepper and salt free seasoning as desired. Enjoy!

Cilantro Lime Tilapia Tacos

Nutritional info: 427 calories, 35 g protein, 45 g carbohydrates, 12 g total fat, 142 mg sodium

Servings: 4

Ingredients

2 jalapeno peppers- chopped (if you want less heat)

1 cup shredded cabbage

3 tablespoons lime juice

1 small onion- chopped

4 cloves garlic- finely minced

1 teaspoon olive oil

8 5-inch white corn tortillas

1 pound tilapia filets- rinsed and patted dry

¼ cup fresh cilantro- chopped

Salt and pepper to taste

1 medium avocado- sliced into 8 slices

Lime wedges and fresh chopped cilantro for garnish

2 cups diced tomatoes

4 tablespoons low-fat or fat free sour cream (optional)

Instructions

Add olive oil to a skillet and heat.

Add in the onions and sauté them until caramelized then add in the garlic and mix well.

Add the tilapia into the skillet and cook it until the flesh begins to flake.

Add in the tomatoes, lime juice, jalapeno peppers and cilantro and cook over medium high heat for 5 minutes before you break up the fish and get everything combined perfectly.

Season as desired with pepper and salt.

Now heat the tortillas for few minutes on each side in a skillet to make them warm.

Serve ¼ cup of the fish on every warmed tortilla together with 2 slices of avocado.

Divide ¼ cup of the shredded cabbage and a tablespoon of fat free or low fat sour cream (totally optional) between the tacos.

Garnish with a fresh dash of cilantro and some lime wedges.

Stuffed Delicata Squash

Nutritional info: 318 calories, 14.0 g fat, 35.0 g carbohydrates; 18.0 g protein, 480 mg sodium

Servings: 4

Ingredients

½ cup low-fat plain or nonfat yogurt

6 teaspoons extra-virgin olive oil- divided

½ teaspoon salt- divided

4 teaspoons of toasted pepitas (see Tip)

2 tablespoons chili powder

½ cup bulgur

8 ounces of lean ground beef- (at 90% or leaner)

1 cup water

1 small onion- chopped

2 small delicata squash (about 12 ounces each) - halved and seeded

Instructions

Preheat your oven to 425 degrees F.

Use 2 teaspoons of oil to brush the sides of the squash that are cut and sprinkle on top ¼ teaspoon of salt.

Place the squash face down onto a large baking sheet and bake them until a bit browned on the edges and tender, for 25 to 30 minutes.

As the squash bakes, bring the water and the bulgur to a boil in a small sauce pan. Lower the heat and cover and allow it to simmer until tender and a lot of the liquid is absorbed (for about 10 minutes) then drain once done.

Heat the rest of the oil over medium heat in a large skillet.

Add in the onions and cook for 4 to 5 minutes as you stir until they begin to brown.

Add in the chilli powder, beef and the remaining quarter tablespoon of salt and let it cook as you stir and break up any chunks using a spoon for about 5 minutes until the meat is cooked all the way through.

Add in the bulgur and stir and cook for 1 more minute. Add in the yogurt and stir it in.

Spoon ¾ of the filling and add it into each half of the squash. Serve it sprinkled with some pepitas.

Tip: To get the best flavor, toast some chopped seeds or nuts. Place a dry skillet over medium low heat. Once it heats, add in the nuts or seeds and cook as you stir occasionally for 2 to 4 minutes, until fragrant.

Line your baking sheets with foil to keep them in great shape and to catch any accidental spills or drips.

Healthy Pasta Salad

Nutritional info: 387.19 calories, 254mg sodium, 18g protein, 46g carbs, 15g fat

Servings: 4

Ingredients

1 cup fresh mozzarella- chopped

¼ cup pine nuts- toasted

4 cups whole wheat penne pasta

Pinch of sea salt

1 bunch fresh basil- coarsely chopped

4 tablespoon extra-virgin olive oil

2 cups cherry tomatoes- halved

⅛ teaspoon cracked black pepper

Instructions

Add water to a large pot and bring it to a boil.

Add a drizzle of some olive oil to make sure the pasta doesn't stick to the pot. Add in the pasta to the pot of boiling water and cook until al dente for 8 to 10 minutes string only once. Sieve the pasta.

For the pine nuts, place a large fat plan over medium high heat and add in the pine nuts to toast.

Add them in and cook as you stir repeatedly to avoid burning them. Toast until the nuts smell buttery and are light brown for about 2 minutes.

Take them out of the pan right away. Toss the cooked pasta in a large bowl together with the rest of the ingredients.

The warm pasta is bound to melt the cheese slightly. Enjoy!

Conclusion

Thank you again for downloading this book!

I hope this book was able to help you to understand how to lose weight, fight heart disease and hypertension by following the DASH diet.

The next step is to implement what you have learnt.

SUBSCRIBE to get the FREE Life Starter E-book! Having a hard time staying committed to things, always finding your self dabbling, find out how to stop that along with tons more. We also left multiple bonuses in the book that can change your life forever! =➔http://eepurl.com/cvrH5r

Lastly SUBSCRIBE to this link to never miss out on FREE, and .99-cent book offers! ==➔http://eepurl.com/cxzVpH

Finally, if you enjoyed this book, would you be kind enough to leave a review for this book on Amazon?

Click here to leave a review for this book on Amazon!

https://www.amazon.com/dp/B01MZGCWAD

Thank you and good luck!